101 Fast And Natural Weight Loss Tips

101 Fast And Natural Weight Loss Tips
by **Jaime Carlyle**

Printed in the United States of America

Copyright © 2010 **Jaime Carlyle**

Contents

Introduction

The Good Old Days...

There was a time in this world when the need to lose weight was completely unheard of. People ate well, but they worked well too. They woke up early in the morning and then engaged in a whole day's work. This work was mostly physical labor. People worked in fields digging, sowing, harvesting. They tilled the soil, rode horses, worked on farms and ranches. The result was that they could afford to eat almost anything they wanted in whatever quantities they wanted.

But that was ages ago. The world has changed so much since those days. Life styles have changed so much and the comforts and facilities have increased so much. But every rose has its thorn. As a result of all these comforts and amenities the state of physical well being has really changed. Most of us have sedentary jobs that demand little or no exercise at all. To put it simply, things have become so damn easy. And just as can be expected, weight gain has become a major concern for almost every city dweller.

During the period of thoughtless youth it is not such a major concern. The young practically eat nothing and so weight problems do not bother them so much. But as soon as you turn twenty, you start showing signs of weight gain and in all the wrong places.

It is not about the hour glass figure or the perfectly sculpted and toned body. It is more about staying fit and remaining healthy to ensure a long, disease free life. Every body knows that those extra pounds spell illness. All over the world people are switching to a healthier life style and the catch line is indeed weight loss.

This book is dedicated solely to the cause of losing weight and that too in the most surprising ways you ever heard of. There is only one thing that you have to bear in mind. Weight loss does not happen by itself. There are only two ways to accomplish it...

101 Fast And Natural Weight Loss Tips

The first is by watching what you eat and the second is by seeing to it that your body gets the exercise that it needs.

As you go through the following pages, my hope is that you are continually amazed by all the "everyday" things you can be doing to lose 10 pounds...or more.

101 Fast And Natural Weight Loss Tips

Chapter 1

101 Tips To Lose Weight

1.

Drink plenty of water. Our bodies need a lot of water so give in to water. Water is not just a way to flush out toxins but if you have more water in your body you will generally feel healthier and fitter. This it self will discourage any tendency to gorge. The best thing about water is that is has no calories at all.

2.

Start your day with a glass of water. As soon as you wake up, gulp down a glass of cool water. It is a wonderful way to start your day and you only need a lesser quantity of your breakfast drink after that. A glass of water lets out all your digestive juices and sort of lubricates the insides of your body. You may have your morning cup of tea but have it after a glass of water. It is good for you.

3.

Drink a glass of water before you start the meal. Water naturally needs some space so that you feel fuller without actually having to stuff yourself.

4.

Have another glass of water while you are having the meal. Again this is another way of making yourself full so that you can actually rise from the table eating less but feeling full just the same. Instead of drinking it in one gulp, take sips after each morsel. It will help the food to settle faster so that you get that feeling that you are full faster.

5.

Stay away from sweetened bottle drinks, especially sodas. All those colas and fizzy drinks are sweetened with sugar and sugar means calories. The more you can cut out on these sweetened bottle drinks, the better for you. So if you must drink sodas, then stick to diet sodas.

6.

Include in your diet things that contain more water like tomatoes and watermelons. These things contain 90 to 95 % water so that there is nothing that you have to lose by feasting on them. They fill you up without adding to the pounds.

7.

Eat fresh fruit instead of drinking fruit juice. Juice is often sweetened but fresh fruits have natural sugars. When you eat fruit, you are taking in a lot of fiber, which is needed by the body, and fruits of course are an excellent source of vitamins.

8.

If you do have a craving for fruit juice then go for fresh fruit juice instead of these that contain artificial flavors and colors. Or even better, try making your own fruit juice taking care not to sweeten it with too many calories.

9.

Choose fresh fruit over processed fruits. Processed and canned fruits do not have as much fiber as fresh fruit and processed and canned fruits are nearly always sweetened.

10.

Increase your fiber intake. Like I mentioned, the body needs a lot of fiber. So try to include in your diet as many fruits and vegetables as you can.

11.

Go crazy on vegetables. Vegetables are your best bet when it comes to losing pounds. Nature has a terrific spread when it comes to choosing vegetables. And the leafy green vegetables are your best bet. Try to include a salad in you diet always.

12.

Eat intelligently. The difference between man and beast is that we are driven by intelligence while beasts are driven by instinct. Do not just eat something because you feel like eating it. Ask your self whether your body really needs it.

13.

Watch what you eat. Keep a watchful eye on every thing that goes in. Sometimes the garnishes can be richer than the food itself. Accompaniments too can be very rich. Remember that it is the easiest thing in the world to eat something without realizing that it was something that you should not have eaten. Selective memory you know...

14.

Control that sweet tooth. Remember that sweet things generally mean more calories. It is natural that we have cravings for sweet things especially chocolates and other confectionery. Go easy on these things and each time you consume something sweet understand that it is going to add on somewhere.

15.

Fix times to have meals and stick to it. Try to have food at fixed times of the day. You can stretch these times by half an hour, but anything more than that is going to affect your eating pattern, the result will either be a loss of appetite or that famished feeling which will make you stuff yourself with more than what is required the next time you eat.

16.

Eat only when you are hungry. Some of us have the tendency to eat whenever we see food. We use parties as an excuse to stuff ourselves. Understand that the effect of a whole week of dieting can be wasted by just one day's party food. Whenever you are offered something to eat do not decline it completely but just break off a nibble so that you appear to mind your manners and at the same time can watch your diet.

17.

Quit snacking in between meals. Do not fall for snacks in between meals. This is especially true for those who have to travel a lot. They feel that the only time they can get a bite to eat is snacks and junk food. The main problem with most snacks and junk food is that they are usually less filling and contain a lot of fat and calories. Just think about French fries...tempting but terribly fattening.

18.

Snack on vegetables if you must. You might get the pangs of hunger in between meals. It is something that you can very well control. Or even better, try munching on carrots. They are an excellent way to satisfy those hungry pangs and are good for your eyes and teeth. True, you might end up being called Bugs Bunny, but its miles better to be called Bugs Bunny than fatso.

19.

Go easy on tea and coffee. Tea and coffee are harmless by themselves. It is when you add the cream and sugar that they become fattening. Did you know that having a cup of tea or coffee that has cream and at least two cubes of sugar is as bad as having a big piece of rich chocolate cake?

20.

Try to stick to black tea or coffee. Black tea or coffee can actually be good for you. But personally I would like to recommend tea rather than coffee. The caffeine in the coffee is not really good for you because it is an alkaloid and can affect other functions of your body like the metabolism.

21.

Count the calories as you eat. It is a good idea to have an idea of the calories that most food items have. If it is a packaged item then the label is sure to have the calories that the substance has.

22.

Be sure to burn out those extra calories by the end of the week. If you feel that you have consumed more calories than you should have during the week, it happens you know, and then make sure that you work off those extra calories by the end of the week.

23.

Stay away from fried things. Fried things are an absolute no-no. The more fried things that you avoid, the lesser weight you will gain. Fried things are called so because they are fried in oil or fat. And even if the external oil is drained away, there is still a lot of hidden oil in it so stay away from it.

24.

Do not skip meals. The worst thing you can do while watching your diet is skip a meal. It has just the opposite effect of what you want. You need to have at least four regular meals every day.

25.

Fresh vegetables are better than cooked or canned vegetables. Try to eat your vegetables raw. When you cook them, you are in fact taking away nearly half the vitamins in them. And canned vegetables too are processed and are not nearly half as good as fresh vegetables. When you buy your vegetables it would be a good thing to see if the label says that it is pesticide free.

26.

Nothing more than an egg a day. Eggs are not such a bright idea. It would be best to reduce your intake of eggs to maybe three in a week. But for those of you die hard egg fans, you may have up to one egg a day but nothing more than that.

27.

Make chocolates a luxury and not a routine. Chocolates are not or at least they should not be a part of your diet. So do not indulge too much in them. Even the bitter chocolates are not good for you because though the sugar is less there is still the cream in them.

28.

Choose a variety of foods from all food groups every day. This is a fine way of keeping deficiency diseases at bay. Change the items included in your diet every day. This is an excellent way of keeping deficiency diseases at bay and it helps you to experiment with a variety of dishes and there by you do not get bored of your diet.

29.

If you can say no to alcoholic beverages please do. Alcoholic beverages too are not good for you. Beer can be fattening and the rest of the alcoholic drinks may not be fattening by themselves but after a couple of swigs you will be in no position to watch your diet and your appetite too will be something to battle with.

30.

Try to have breakfast within one hour of waking. It's always best to have breakfast within an hour of waking so that your body can charge itself with the energy it needs for the day. The idea is not to wait for your self to get really hungry. Breakfast is the most important meal of the day but that does not mean that it should be the most filling meal of the day.

31.

50 to 55% of your diet should be carbohydrates. It is a myth that you should try and avoid carbohydrates when you are on a diet. Rather the other way round I should say. Carbohydrates are a ready source of energy and so 50 to 55% of your diet should be carbohydrates.

32.

25 to 30% of your diet should be proteins. Various processes and activities are going on in our bodies. Things are broken down and being built up again. Resistance has to be built up, recovery from disease too is needed and for all this the body needs plenty of proteins so see to it that 25 to 30 % of your diet consists of proteins.

33.

Fats should only be 15 to 20 %. You need only this much of fat in your diet so keep it at that.

34.

Try and adopt a vegetarian diet. A vegetarian diet is undoubtedly better for those of us watching our diet. There are a lot of advantages of keeping to a vegetarian diet but I do not want to sing an ode to vegetarianism now. What I would suggest is keep to a vegetarian diet as much as you can. Make a non-vegetarian diet a week end event or something if you find it impossible to give up eating all those animals.

35.

Choose white meat rather than red. White meat, which includes fish and fowl, is miles better than red meat, which includes beef and pork for those trying to lose weight.

36.

High Fiber multigrain breads are better than white breads. Remember how I told you to increase the fiber content in your food; well this is the answer to that. It is not only better in terms of the fiber content but also in terms of the protein content as well.

37.

Reduce your intake of pork. Pork is not something that can help you to lose weight. So the less pork you eat the better chances you have of losing weight. And remember that pork includes the pork products as well, things like bacon, ham and sausages.

38.

Limit your sugar intake. If you cannot have things unsweetened go for sugar substitutes. These things are just as sweetening but are certainly not fattening.

39.

Graze 5 to 6 times a day. Instead of sticking to just three meals a day, try grazing. Grazing means try having 5 or 6 smaller meals instead of three king sized meals. It is an excellent way of having smaller quantities of food.

40.

Go ahead eat cheat food, but only for flavor.
There are many things which you have to avoid
from your diet but which you may have an
undying craving for. Do not avoid them
altogether. You could call them cheat foods and
indulge in them once in a while. But take care
just to tingle your taste buds, do not over do it.
Instead of that share them with others.

41.

Watch your fat intake. Each fat gram contains 9
calories so by reading the total calories on a
food and knowing the quantity of fat, you can
estimate the % of fat, which should in no way
exceed 30% of the food.

42.

Go easy on salt, as too much salt is one of the
causes of obesity. Make it a point to really cut
down on salt. Try to bring down your salt intake
to half of what it was last year.

43.

Change from table butter to cholesterol free butter. If you have a choice why not go for it, any way it is healthier for you and tastes just the same. Bear in mind that these small changes can go a long way towards weight reduction.

44.

Instead of frying things try baking them without fat. Baking is by far a healthier method of preparing food than frying. Baking requires lesser oil or fat.

45.

Use a non stick frying pan for your cooking so that you do not have to add oil. The golden rule is to try and avoid as much oil as possible and a non stick pan is the perfect solution to this problem.

46.

Boil your vegetables instead of cooking them, or even better, eat them fresh. However if you do not like eating your vegetables as it is, try steaming them without adding anything at all. This is probably the healthiest way to eat cabbages, cauliflowers and a host of other vegetables.

47.

Carry parsley with you. Parsley is an excellent thing to munch on in between meals. Not just is it good for you in terms of vitamins, but it is also a perfect way of making your breath fresher.

48.

Choose low fat substitutes or no fat substitutes. There are plenty of low fat or even no fat substitutes available in the market so why not choose wisely. It is much better for your heart too. Many people just go shopping and pick up whatever they can. They do not bother to find out if there are any substitutes for the thing they are looking for.

In the markets of today, you will be astounded at the range of goods that manufacturers have to offer. In fact with all the hue and cry that is being made about weight loss, low fat substitutes and no fat substitutes are hitting the stands faster than mushrooms that sprout after the first rains.

So the next time you head for the stores instead of picking up what you have always picked up, see if there are better substitutes.

Remember that our bodies need nutrients and not just calories. Fats give us nutrients but with more calories than proteins or carbohydrates do.

49.

Avoid crash diets. They are bad for health and you will gain what you have lost once you take a break. Crash diets are not a solution to weight loss. It might seem as if you have lost few pounds but the moment you give up on the crash diet every thing will bounce back with a vengeance.

Take a look at it in this way. Do you think that it is possible for a person to survive on a crash diet for the rest of his or her life? Certainly not! So at some time or the other, you will have to give up the crash diet and then you will see for yourself that a crash diet does more harm than good on the long run.

Crash diets may have a lot to promise, but very rarely do these promises ring true. Crash diets are things people go on in order to wear an old dress or suit for a particular occasion. That is the only purpose that they serve as far as I can see.

50.

God gave us teeth for a reason...

Therefore we should develop a habit of chewing all food including liquid food and soft foods like sweets, ice creams at least 8 to 12 times. This is essential to add saliva to the food, as it is only in the saliva that sugar is digested.

Often we find that whatever goes into our mouth goes down like lightning. We hardly give the saliva any time to act on the food. So does digestion take place like it should? Do we just stuff our tummies with food that does not get digested or in other words that does not yield the benefits that it should?

51.

Dry wine is better than sweet wine. Sweet wines naturally contain a lot of sugar. But on the other hand, in dry wines most of this sugar has been fermented away so from the weight point of view dry wines are better than sweet wines.

52.

When you decide it is time to start working out, start slowly and do not get discouraged if you do not achieve your fitness goals after the first week. Many people make this mistake. They feel that if they really push their bodies they can lose more weight in a couple of work outs. This is a very serious thing in fact.

If you try to push your body too much in the first few goes, you are likely to end up with sprained joints, a sore back and even torn ligaments. The rule to be followed here is slow and steady wins the race.

53.

Check your weight before you start the routine and keep checking for changes but do not expect a radical change immediately, it might be one or two weeks before you notice some change. However it is crucial that you continue to monitor your weight. You may bear in mind the fact that even a few pounds loss is a big achievement.

54.

When you do notice a change, reward yourself. When I say reward I do not mean go for some goodies like chocolates or sweets. Maybe you could go for a movie or buy yourself something like a new dress or a trinket.

This is something that can keep you going. It is a good idea to save on the money that you wanted to spend on ice creams and chocolates and then treat your self to something more substantial.

55.

You can take a day off from exercise every week. This is not just a very good idea but it is part of the exercise routine. Your body needs a day off from an exercise routine so do not hesitate to take a day off from what ever you have been doing.

56.

Exercise out doors as much as possible. There are two advantages of doing whatever you are doing out side. One advantage is that it gives your body a chance to get a lot of the much needed fresh air and sunshine.

The second advantage is that the surroundings keep you perked up and it is a break from remaining cooped up all day long

57.

Try to collect some information about exercise, there are a lot of things that you can do at home. Extensive research has been done on exercise and plenty of this information is easily available.

You can try browsing the internet or getting a book or two on how to exercise at home. This information will be useful to you to know how much you need to work out on each specific exercise in order to burn off the desired number of calories.

58.

Try to get somebody to exercise along with you. But it should be somebody committed or else your interest might dwindle. This is indeed an excellent idea. One of the advantages of getting a committed person to exercise with you is that it keeps you going.

There may be days when you feel just too lazy to crawl out of bed in the mornings. On such days, the knowledge that some body is waiting for you is enough to slide out of bed.

Another advantage is that you can discuss your progress and fears with another person and be a sympathetic listener to the other person as well. This is a fine way of getting motivated your self.

59.

Stop when your body has had enough. There is no sense in pushing it. When you have worked out for a considerable time, your body will start giving you signals.

Heed those signals. This is particularly true in the initial stages. Take one step at a time. Stop when you are out of breath or when a certain part of your body tells you that it has had enough.

60.

If you want to increase your time of exercise or your work out routine, do it gradually and not in sudden steps.

Well easier said than done. Most of us have such hectic schedules that it is quite impossible to fit in time for exercise right? Wrong. I want to say it once and for all, your body, or anybody's body for that matter needs proper exercise. If you make up your mind to do it, you just can.

61.

Select an exercise pattern to suit your life style. All of us have different life styles and professions so there is no sense in trying to follow the book strictly. Try and follow an exercise routine that is suitable for you. You have to understand that even more important than the exercise itself is sticking to it. So unless you choose something that can suit your life style, you are not going to stick to it.

62.

Do not stand, walk. If you can walk about then do so. Do not stand in a fixed position. Pacing about is a good thing to do. If you are thinking deeply about something, try pacing about, it will aid in your thinking.

63.

Do not sit, stand. If you can stand, then do not sit. The golden rule is to choose a position that is less comfortable.

64.

Do not lie down, sit. The rule that we mentioned above rings true here as well.

65.

Do not be a couch potato. It is the easiest thing in the world to become a couch potato. You know what we are talking about don't you? That shapeless thing that sits or reclines on a shapeless chair in front of the television and stupidly munches away at something fried!

If you are inclined to become a promising old couch potato, break the habit, cut at the very root of the vine. And you want to know what is the best way for that? Take away that favorite chair of yours. In fact, it would be a very good idea if you could keep a chair that is not too comfortable in front of the TV.

This will discourage any tendency to become a couch potato.

66.

If you have a sitting job, stand up and stretch yourself every half an hour. Most of the jobs today are indeed sitting jobs that are in one word sedentary. This is especially true for those who sit and punch away at the keyboard or toy with the mouse all day long.

So if you have such a job, make it a point to get up at least every half an hour and stretch your self.

67.

While making telephone calls try walking up and down. I hope you will agree with me that this is an excellent suggestion.

68.

Use the stairs instead of the elevator whenever you can. Elevators are one hell of a convenience particularly if you have to go up or down some twenty floors. But elevators also make us very lazy.

There may be no sense in trudging up some twenty flights of stairs because by the time you get there you will be totally pooped. But while coming down, if you have the time, you can easily come down the stairs instead of using the elevator. Coming down is not at all exhausting.

And talking about the time factor, I don't think that there is much of a difference. Sometimes waiting for an elevator door to open at your floor after you hit the button can take up all of eternity.

69.

Smoking is bad for weight loss. Smoking as such may not contribute to weight loss but smoking leads to other conditions like erratic eating habits and excessive dependence on things like coffee.

70.

If you hate running, remember, you do not have to run a marathon to stay fit. 10 minutes of cardio each day is good enough for most.

71.

And if you cannot run, try walking. 15 minutes of brisk walking a day is enough to keep most fit.

72.

Any distance is walkable if you have the time, so consider walking to places that you would normally drive (such as work or the market if they are not too far away). It may take you longer, but the health benefits will last you a lifetime.

73.

It sounds strange, but some people have reported that they lost more weight when they drank black coffee before a workout. While there is no hard data to support this, nutritionists speculate that the caffeine in coffee makes the body rely more on fat for fuel during the work out. It is worth trying!

74.

Here is a corollary to the tip above: Avoid drinking coffee in excess, as it tends to desensitize your body to the fat burning effects of caffeine.

75.

Stop using remote controls. Remote controls are the bane of a prospective weight loser. They may be remarkable gadgets by themselves but from the weight loss point of view, they just are not very helpful.

They really encourage us to take a laid back kind of attitude towards life itself. In fact if remote controls were not there, the television would not have become so popular. It is because of remote controls that people can remain where they are and switch from one channel to the other. And they only have to twitch a finger muscle to achieve this.

Now, I have nothing against multi channel television sets but what I strongly advocate is that you get up from where you are and change the channel of the TV each time you want to do so.

The same thing holds true for other remote controls as well. As it is we have remote controlled TVs, DVD players, A/Cs, garage doors, gateways and what not. The next thing we know is that we will have remote controlled people as well.

76.

Do things like fetching, turning things off and on by yourself. Often when we come back tired from work, we tend to get others to do simple chores for us. These things are no big deal. They are things that we can very well do for our selves but we do not.

That is why we often ask our kids to fetch us this or take away that.

Training your pet is a wonderful thing indeed. It is quite remarkable how some people get their dogs to fetch them something. But the fact is that while you may be making sure that your dog is getting a lot of exercise, you are neglecting your bit of the story.

77.

Here's a pop quiz. Escalators help us to:

1.   Move up and down faster
2.   Gain weight
3.   Stand stupidly as they move up and down
4.   Look down at other people when you are going down
5.   Look up to others when we are going up

You have to pick the correct answer from the 5 alternatives given. You can see for your self that all the options are in a way correct. So the next time you travel on an escalator, do not just stand there...climb up or down along with it. (Or better yet, take the stairs.)

78.

During commercial breaks walk about. If you want to sit all evening with your eyes glued to the tube, then do so. But at least spare your eyes the agony of a commercial break.

When the next commercial flashes on screen, instead of surfing, get up and take a walk. Reach over and try to touch your toes or do any such simple exercise that will at least get the blood flowing in your veins.

79.

Wriggle your toes and your fingers whenever you can. This too is a stress buster and it gives you a chance to at least work your hand and leg joints. This will tell you how sore they are and if their condition is so bad, just think of the rest of your body.

80.

Turn on music and dance like wild. Let your hair down once in a while. Go back to the days of wild child hood. Close the door of your room, turn on your sound system to the highest volume possible (but a little lower than the level at which your neighbors start to complain) and then do the wackiest dance that you can think of. Jump on your bed and jump off it again.

Roll all over the floor. Pretend that you are Michael Jackson or Madonna (you will never see them keeping still) and do every boogie move that you know.

81.

Carry a soft flying disc or Frisbee with you. Toss it around and get up to fetch it. This is also an excellent way to beat stress. It makes a person feel good to throw something away forcefully when the person is all worked up. And the thing that you throw is something soft and cannot damage anything, then what is stopping you?

It is not really the throwing part that we are interested in. It is the fetching part. Each time you get up to fetch it back; you are giving yourself a chance to stretch those muscles and joints

82.

Get off the bus a block before your destination and walk the rest of the way. You might not have time to fit in long walks in your busy schedule so this is one way of ensuring that you at least get to walk for a little bit every day. If you take the bus or the subway, get down at an earlier station and see if you can walk the rest of the way.

If you drive to work, see if you can get space in a parking lot that is a little away from your office.

83.

When nobody is watching try doing pelvic gyrations. If you take a moment to observe it you will see that it is the mid section of our body that gets the least bit of exercise and that is probably why the signs of weight gain are mostly seen there.

It is the same reason why we find it very difficult to lose weight in that section. So the best thing that you can do is consciously try to give that part a little bit of exercise.

Stomach crunches might be too strenuous an exercise to start off with but gyrations are relatively mild. Pelvic gyrations make you thrust your midsection towards all directions and this is the best way of tightening every muscle in that mid section and that is of course what weight loss is all about.

84.

Tuck in your tummy whenever you walk. Get that proper gait. And the best way for that is to tuck in your tummy and inflate your chest. Do not let your tummy hang above your belt line like some unruly layer of flesh. Bring it under the belt.

Each time you tuck in your tummy, you will feel the pressure on the muscles of your stomach. This tightening and loosening of these muscles is even better than stomach crunches.

85.

Try breathing exercises. You might be surprised to know that breathing exercises too can lead to weight loss. If you are doing the breathing exercises properly, you will find that you can exert a lot of pressure on the muscles around the mid section.

You can feel a tightening of these muscles each time you breathe in or breathe out. So go ahead and breathe properly, it is good for you.

86.

Try yoga. Yoga is one of the best ways of losing weight. Of course I cannot go into a full lecture about yoga but I can tell you that I have never seen people with better-toned bodies than those who practice yoga.

One of the benefits of yoga is that you learn to control virtually every muscle and joint of your body so that the issue of weight gain will cease to exist.

87.

Try massaging your partner. This is a fun way to lose weight. It is something that can give your partner a lot of pleasure and at the same time can give you a lot of exertion there by leading to weight loss.

The attitude should of course be you scratch my back I will scratch yours. It should not be a one sided effort or else the interest will soon dwindle.

In fact it is a good idea if couples take up weight loss routines together. They can keep watch over each other, help control those urges to eat and motivate each other to stick to the routine.

There are a lot of things that couples can do together that can help them to keep physically active.

88.

If you cannot think of any thing else to do try punching your pillow. Now here is another one of those weird ideas but believe me it works. Not too many of us have punching bags at home and if you have a really fluffy pillow giving it a good punching routine is just as good as anything else.

This is also a nice way of letting off steam so go for it. After all something is better than nothing. But I would suggest that you do not hit it too violently or else the stuffing might come out. Do not bother too much about the force with which you hit the pillow. It is number of hits that are important. Try to get at least fifty punches in one bout.

I would like to give you a little tip. If there is somebody that you particularly dislike like your boss or your neighbor, or may be your ex boy friend or girl friend, try fixing a picture of the persons head on the top of your pillow and then try punching it. I promise you, it will give you a lot of satisfaction.

89.

Instead of waddling up and down the staircase, try taking them two at a time. Now this is something that you have to be careful about because we do not want you to trip. So when you do this make sure that your feet are well and truly planted on each step before you increase the beat and try two at a time.

90.

If you have a dog, take it for a run and let the dog lead you on. You will be surprised as to how much exercise a dog can give you.

Animals are sensible enough to know that they need a lot of exercise so let your animal lead you on. Take your pet dog out for a walk and before you know what hit you, it will turn out to be a run.

91.

Join a dance class. Dancing is a wonderful way to burn off those extra calories. It is true. When you dance you are in fact burning away a lot of calories. Of course we are not referring to the slow ballroom kind of dances in which one person actually leans on the other one for support. We are talking about fast dances.

The best way to do it is by joining a dance class because they will really wok you out. But I would suggest that you wait for a couple more pounds to vanish before you think of becoming a ballerina.

92.

Whenever you can, lean against a wall with your hands flattened against the wall and in such a way that your face is very close to the wall. Then use your hands to push your body away from the wall. Do this two or three times at a stretch.

93.

If there is a pool nearby go for swims as often as you can, swimming is one of the best exercises. Water has a lot of advantages. And if nothing else, a cool dip in a pool is a wonderful stress reliever.

94.

Try playing something like table tennis or basket ball. Games are a fun way to lose weight. It is much more exciting to play a game than just work out by yourself. The best thing about games is that they are addictive. Once you start playing you will soon end up with a friends' circle and then the playing goes on without even you knowing it.

It is something that you can look forward to and there is no stress involved in this program. In fact the more you play the less you will consider this to be a part of your weight loss program. As you burn away those calories, you will also be able to expand your social circle.

95.

Any work out should start with a 5 to 10 minute warm up and should end with a 5 to 10 minute cool down session. Whatever physical exercise you are involved in, you must remember to warm up before the exercise really starts. Do not just plunge into the water and start thrashing about, to put it figuratively.

Your body needs to reach a certain level of readiness before it can actually start responding to exercise. And this readiness is achieved by the warming up process.

96.

Do not carry your mobile phone around but leave it in a place where you can hear it ringing. In this way you make sure that you at least get up and walk towards it. This might sound silly but I really mean it. You need a reason to keep yourself going.

Life today has become so easy that we have every thing at our fingertips. All we have to do is push a button here and push a button there. The only things that get any exercise at all are our fingers. Years ago Charles Darwin put forward a theory of use and disuse.

According to this theory, a certain part of the body that is put to constant use develops a lot and a certain part of the body that has no use at all becomes smaller and smaller and gradually ceases to exist.

Certain examples that he quoted were the long neck of the giraffe, which appeared to become longer and longer when the giraffe stretched higher and higher to reach the leaves at the treetops. He quoted the example of the absence of a tail in human beings to illustrate the example of the theory of disuse.

101 Fast And Natural Weight Loss Tips

Now if Darwin's theory were to prove true, as the years go by man is likely to end up with just a huge head, a few fingers and maybe some other parts of the body that are also put to use.

That is why I made it a point to say that you have to drive your self to move about. A cell phone may be convenient, but the same thing can turn out to simplify life just a little too bit. There are other arguments against the use of cell phones but that is beside our topic.

What I would suggest is that at home or in your office, leave the cell phone lying about so that you can hear it ring, but cannot just reach into your pocket and answer it. See to it that you have to actually stand up and walk a few steps before you can pick it up.

97.

While traveling in an elevator instead of just standing there and staring stupidly at the numbers going up or down, try raising your self onto your toes and then back on your feet again. Do this several times. Also try flexing your buttock muscles as well.

In fact there are many muscles in our body that we can twitch and flex without inviting the attention of others. Even if others do notice you, its no big deal provided you are flexing a muscle in a decent part of the body. (Most of the other parts do not have muscles any way.) Others might brand you as a health freak but it is miles better to be known as a heath freak than as a sack of potatoes.

98.

Undress and stare at yourself in front of your mirror. If what you see displeases you, then you have all the more reason to work out. Try tucking in the extra fat in all those wide areas, this will give you an idea of which part you need to be working on.

Turn to your side and get a very good view of your side profile. This is an excellent way of checking whether you have a tummy that is starting to bulge or has bulged already.

Try pulling in air and then take a look at your tummy, if it has gone in even a little bit, there is hope for you. If you start now, you can control it where it is now and may be if you really set your mind to it, you can lose a couple of inches in a just a few weeks.

Weighing your self on your bathroom scales is a good idea but personally I would recommend this mirror viewing. To be very frank, a few pounds gain may shock you but does not really disgust you. But a flabby figure and extra fat certainly will.

99.

If you have a banister rail or a balustrade that will support you, sit on it and pump your legs as if you are riding a bicycle, taking care not to fall off of course.

This might sound like another crazy idea and I don't want to argue with you about that. I just want to tell you that by doing such crazy things, you are in fact not missing a single chance to lose those extra pounds. It is a way of keeping your mind alert all the time. Every thing must look like an opportunity to you.

100.

Do not slouch in your chair but try to maintain an erect posture with your tummy tucked in. Slouching is a very bad habit. Not only is it bad for your back but it also gives you a very flabby figure. It is your way of saying yes to a comfortable, weight-gaining pose.

Make it a point to always sit as erect as you can. It is also a terrific way to ward off back problems.

101.

Psst. I would like to let you in on a secret. As it is I understand that most of us tend to put on weight particularly in the mid section, right. It is the tummy that seems to have a mind of its own. Well I will tell you a sure shot method to reduce the flab around the waist line. Mind you this does not hold true for post pregnancy tummies. This is what you have to do.

Breathe in air as strongly as you can and as you do so, tuck in your tummy as much as you can. Hold it like this for a few seconds and then slowly release your breath taking care not to let out your tummy. Try to keep breathing like this at least fifty or sixty times in a day.

In fact breathe like this whenever you can remember to do so. After the first day, you should feel the muscles of your stomach tightening each time you do this. Then you know that you are on the right track. If you practice this without fail for 20 days, at the end of the twentieth day, you will have lost at least an inch.

Below I have included a table of the various exercises and the number of calories that can

101 Fast And Natural Weight Loss Tips

be burnt with each exercise. Choose what you can do best and choose something that you will enjoy doing in the long run as well.

The choice of the exercise is completely left to you but try to do whatever you wish to do for at least twenty minutes. It is only after you do the exercise for twenty minutes that the actual calorie burning sets in.

Aerobics	200-250 calories
Bicycling, Stationary	250-300 calories
Bicycling, Actual	300-400 calories
Running, 5-6 mph	300-350 calories
Stair climber	200-250 calories
Swimming laps	350 calories
Walking briskly	150-180 calories

101 Fast And Natural Weight Loss Tips

From this you can see for yourself that walking is not at all something that has to be sidelined. If you really find your days to be too full to fit in any other form of exercise, then walking is your best bet. Walk as much as you can.

Try getting to places and leaving places a little early. This will give you time to walk.

Get rid of those extra calories and pounds as early as you can and try to enjoy life the best you can without inviting all those terrible diseases that come with a few extra pounds.

Chapter 2

Understanding Your Body: A Different Perspective

It is strange how the secrets that we try so hard to find out have already been discovered ages ago and that too in the most unlikely places and by the most unlikely people. People who lived ages ago in the East have already solved many of the puzzles of the human body.

101 Fast And Natural Weight Loss Tips

The Indian system of medicine, which is called Ayurveda, is a wonder in itself. The explanations in this stream of science at first glance may seem far-fetched but when you really sit down and think about it, you will be astounded by the knowledge and understanding that the ancient Indian sages had. I have included a little bit on the Indian system of medicine that is particular to the subject of our interest, that is the diet and its control.

Take time to go through the stream of thought in the following pages, it is more than interesting.

Chapter 3

How Much Do You Know?

I have included a simple test to see how much you have grasped about the proper way to control your diet. Go ahead and do the test, you might find it interesting.

1) Which of the following is suitable for a between meal snack?

    a) Cheese
    b) Carrots
    c) Yogurt
    d) Coffee
    e) Candy

101 Fast And Natural Weight Loss Tips

2) How many glasses of water should a person have in a day?

    a) 5-6
    b) 10-20
    c) 10- 12
    d) 4-5
    e) 15-20

3) Which of the following is bad as far as weight control is concerned?

    a) snacking
    b) smoking
    c) coffee
    d) crash diets
    e) all the above

4) How many hours sleep does an adult need?

    a) 7-8
    b) 6-7
    c) 8-9
    d) 5-6
    e) 9-10

101 Fast And Natural Weight Loss Tips

5)   Which is better for a person on a diet?

   a)   fresh fruit
   b)   canned fruit
   c)   fruit juice
   d)   processed fruit
   e)   cooked fruit

6)   Which of the following should you always include in your diet?

   a)   nuts
   b)   dried fruits
   c)   fruit juice
   d)   salads
   e)   tea

7)   Which of these two is better for your health?

   a)   coffee
   b)   tea

101 Fast And Natural Weight Loss Tips

8)   The most important meal of the day is

    a)   supper
    b)   snacks
    c)   break fast
    d)   lunch
    e)   tea

9)   Which of the following can you afford to cut out from your diet?

    a)   fats
    b)   carbohydrates
    c)   vegetables
    d)   proteins
    e)   vitamins

10) Which meat is better for health?

    a)   white meat
    b)   red meat
    c)   raw meat

101 Fast And Natural Weight Loss Tips

Answers:

1.   b
2.   c
3.   e
4.   a
5.   a
6.   d
7.   b
8.   c
9.   a
10.   a

101 Fast And Natural Weight Loss Tips

Chapter 4

Muscle Power

Use your brains to answer the test on the best ways to work out.

1) Which is the best exercise among the following?

    a) horse riding
    b) walking
    c) swimming
    d) running
    e) bowling

101 Fast And Natural Weight Loss Tips

2)   Before you need to work out, you need to

   a)   drink water
   b)   warm up
   c)   consult a trainer
   d)   make up your mind
   e)   cool off

 3)   You can afford to take a day off from your
work out every week

   a)   true
   b)   false

4)   Yoga does not help to reduce weight

   a)   true
   b)   false

5)   Breathing exercises strengthen the
      shoulder muscles

   a)   true
   b)   false

101 Fast And Natural Weight Loss Tips

Answers:

1. c
2. b
3. a
4. a
5. b

101 Fast And Natural Weight Loss Tips

Chapter 5

The Starting Point

The enormous amount of excess fat in the human body has made the keyword 'weight loss programs' an instant hit among the common man. No wonder, most of the search engine spiders get a lot of inquiries on this word and the related key words, day in and day out.

Let us dig out the prime reasons behind this problem. It is a matter beyond dispute that there is a direct relation between the food we eat and the weight that adds up. Hence almost all weight loss programs concentrate on making some control on the 'quality' and the 'quantity' on the food we consume.

101 Fast And Natural Weight Loss Tips

Where should we start? Now that you have decided to lose some weight we must of course find an answer to the above question. Let me make it clear that there is no better place than our mind.

We should have a strong resolve towards our aim. Conceive this as a just war towards your good health. As in any war there will be at least one enemy. Here your main enemy would be the basic urge to stuff your self with all the wrong things

Chapter 6

Knowing Our Stomach and Body

Will you be able to find another person exactly like you? If the answer is "No," what made you think that every person's stomach behaves in the same way, accepting all the inputs in the same fashion. This is a basic mistake we often make.

Believe me, your stomach may not be behaving in the same way as your friend's stomach does to a particular food item, be it a chicken piece or a burger. We must know that a particular food, which may be good for certain people, may not be suitable for others. Haven't you heard the proverb, what is wine for Paul may be venom for Peter.

101 Fast And Natural Weight Loss Tips

The Indian system of Ayurveda and yoga is considered as the best way to explain the different types of body nature. The basic constituents are classified as five elements.

Chapter 7

Five Elements:

Earth: All life forces become inert and inactive in this element and more energy is used to keep it active. People with more weight, flesh, fat etc. are good example of predominance of this earth matter in their body. They do not show any anxiety and are not eager to acquire anything, they try to keep away from conflict and their life is moving slowly. When there is a disorder of this element in the body people become selfish and get attached to selfish enjoyments. It is a neutral element.

Water: It keeps the flow of body and life. But it has a natural tendency to cool down. As there is more than 70% water in the body it plays a very important role in the maintenance of heat and circulation of blood etc. It is a negative element.

Fire: It is creating fire in the body – heats the water. It regulates sight, provides strength to the body by digesting the food, induces hunger and thirst, and also maintains suppleness of muscles and beauty of complexion. It helps thinking and facilitates the discrimination power of the brain. It helps production of antibodies.

In short it is the starter of our body-car. Defects in the same causes anemia, jaundice and other digestive problems, and also causes fainting, epilepsy, derangement of brain besides diminishing eyesight and causing growth of cataract in the eyes, it produces acidity and also creates skin problems and de-pigmentation.

That is why great importance is given in eastern therapies to control and preserve the element of fire. It is a positive element.

Air: Air is life itself. It is the strength and conducts every part of our body. It regulates the function of heart, circulation of blood and maintains balance of the body.

It helps respiration and downward movement of stools and urine. It produces sound. Nourishes mental faculties and also the faculty of memory. It moves bile and phlegm, which cannot move in the body by themselves. It is a positive element.

Space: In order for air to circulate in the body and maintain a proper balance, there has to be space. If such circulation is blocked, it creates pain even leading to heart attack, paralysis, fainting etc. It is a negative element.

101 Fast And Natural Weight Loss Tips

Chapter 8

Prakruti – Type – Different Combination of Elements In the Body

If these five basic elements are maintained in proper proportion in the body, a proper metabolism is ensured and the body remains healthy. However due to heredity, eating and living habits more often than not, we disturb one or two of these elements and thus upset the metabolism and there is a predominance of three different types of combinations. Such combination of these elements decide our types-prakrutis. Ayurveda, the Indian medical therapy, has divided people into three types:

101 Fast And Natural Weight Loss Tips

1) Combination through excess of Earth +Water

2) Combination through excess of Fire + Air, and

3)   Excess of Air element

This therapy advocates that while treating the patients, one must keep in mind their respective types. For those people having kapha prakruthi, milk will only create problems.

People, therefore, having bronchitis or asthma indigestion should avoid milk. For people with pitt prakruti, spicy food will enhance their problem. Therefore, what is good for one type could be harmful to another.

Kapha Prakruti: It is a combination of earth and water. These elements occupy the major portion of our body. Sweet foods and drinks when properly digested are reduced to saline and the blood becomes alkaline.

It sustains the body system, increases vigor and there is a marked growth of happiness. It lubricates the joints of bones and keeps them working properly. However, this is possible when there is proper element of fire – heat in the body.

However because of lack of exercise, overheating, eating between the meals when not hungry, eating more indigestible foods like concentrated sweet-fried things causes problems of indigestion and fail to produce enough heat in the body.

This leads to increase in water content and reduction of heat in the body, resulting in problems like dullness, heaviness, increase in fats, common cold bronchitis and later on asthma, arthritis rheumatism etc.

The best way to cure the above ailments of kapha prakruti is to reduce the intake of undesirable foods, cold drinks and foods that only aggravate the problems. They should eat only light digestible food when hungry; avoid sleeping during the day and over sex. Even milk is harmful to them. They should also take physical exercises.

Pitta Prakruti: It is a combination of fire+ air. Excess of heat damages the working of brain – leads to acidity – ulcer, cold due to heat, skin problems, even sexual weakness, short temper and falling out of hair.

101 Fast And Natural Weight Loss Tips

Now, in modern times more anxiety – worries- eating more of fried and spicy foods- more exposure to sun, excessive use of antibiotics indulged in by people increases their problem. It is, therefore essential to avoid these habits as much as possible.

They should take sweet fruit juice as the first thing in the morning and have more fruits, sweet desserts after eating and drink more green juice.

Air Vayu Prakruti: This condition prevails when there is an excess of the element of air. People belonging to this category are more talkative and have day dreams. They need more sleep and have more gas trouble. These imbalances lead to fainting.

The tendency to eat heavy-oily foods- like fried and foods made out of gram etc. increases this tendency. People in such condition should avoid constipation and sleeping during day time, have more physical exercise so as to increase heat and circulation and should avoid unsuitable foods.

Chapter 9

Productive Cycle Controlling Cycle

Basically all the elements in your body should remain in proper proportion-which is called the Metabolism of the body. Any disturbance-excess or less of one element leads to disturbance in other element and becomes the root cause of the disease.

Everyone should try and find out the category and type he or she belongs to and avoid as far as possible those items, which will only aggravate their problems. They should consume food that will suit their type. It may be noted that each and every person is different from the other.

101 Fast And Natural Weight Loss Tips

So there are tendencies and problems of health. But with proper changes in the diet good health can be maintained. The cerebral spinal fluid is produced from the blood and so imbalance in blood of these basic elements leads to imbalance even in cerebral spinal fluid. More salt in food for instance increases the sodium chloride in cerebral spinal fluid, which leads to high blood pressure, etc.

Moreover, the climate plays an important role in its effect on the body. In summer and hot climate, for instance, buttermilk will be useful, but not in winter. Therefore in winter buttermilk should be warmed and black pepper and ginger should be added to it before drinking.

Nature grows the required vegetables and fruits etc. suitable for the nourishment of the body in all different areas and season. So wherever possible locally produced seasonal fruits and vegetable should be eaten.

101 Fast And Natural Weight Loss Tips

Moreover nature also produces several varieties of fruits resembling the shapes of the organs of our body and they are useful and beneficial to that organ.

Apricot	=	Brain
Mango-Papaya	=	Stomach
Almonds	=	Eyes
Apple	=	Heart
Grapes	=	Lunges
Cashew nuts	=	Kidney

Kidney beans (Ripe: Outside skin black)

People belonging to one type or the other type of prakruti (characteristics) can easily find out and eat foods which would do them good and reject foods that will aggravate their problem-tendency.

This practice will also enable us to prevent wasting our energy in digesting and expelling these food intakes not suitable for our body.

101 Fast And Natural Weight Loss Tips

Energy: In order that the body and brain can function properly it is necessary to create energy from the five basic elements. That is why we take food and drinks.

The whole cosmos gets the energy from the sun. All types of natural foods, fruits, vegetables, cereals, pulses etc have in them almost equal measure of positive and negative of sun energy. However foods contain positive and negative properties in varying degrees. They can be divided in six tastes of which all foods and drinks are made of:

Bitter	=	Air	+	Space
Sweet	=	Earth	+	Water
Astringent	=	Air	+	Water
Salty	=	Earth	+	Fire
Pungent	=	Air	+	ire
Sour	=	Water	+	Fire

(hot) (as per Charak Samhitha)

101 Fast And Natural Weight Loss Tips

In our daily diet it is necessary to maintain a proper balance in all these six tastes. Surprisingly, Ayurveda- Indian medical science has made elaborate research in all kinds of fruits, vegetables and minerals and has established their after effect on the human system.

When we take foods more of negative types or more of positive types, we create imbalances, leading to diseases. The body tries to balance the positive and negative excesses in the system and such efforts are called disease.

Surprisingly China has made in depth research for energy derived from food and has come to the conclusion that one should take 65% foods in cereals and pulses like wheat – rice – millet's, grams etc and the balance 35% in milk-milk products, vegetables, dry fruits, oils etc, these would be the ideal contents of a balanced diet.

I am of the opinion that after the body is fully developed one must eat and drink only those things which are suitable to one's body and only when one feels hungry. The fruits and vegetables have in them a natural storage of the sun's energy and if we make a daily practice of having one glass of fruit juice and two or three cups of green juice of vegetables, our requirement for food will be reduced to a minimum and we will have enough energy to maintain the body in a healthy condition.

Please note that care of our digestive system should start from the mouth. Nature has given us teeth to chew. Therefore we should form a habit of chewing all food including liquid food and soft food like sweets, ice-creams, etc. at least 8 to 12 times.

This is necessary to add saliva to the food, for it is only in saliva that the sugar is digested. That is why people eating hastily without chewing and eating more sugar invite diabetes and fat. Chewing less means double work for the stomach. Over-exertion of stomach will invite many diseases and even fat.

Proper chewing gives better taste and satisfaction. Moreover, it enables you to listen to nature's signal that your stomach is full. This in turn enables you to stop eating further. Therefore discussions at the dining table should be avoided as far as possible. Instead, soft music may be played. We should always remember that it is not more quantity or heavy food but the food that is digested gives us energy.

101 Fast And Natural Weight Loss Tips

Diet: The aim of eating and drinking should be to produce enough blood, produce sufficient heat and energy in the body and satisfy the taste.

There are six types of tastes :

1) Sweet

2) Salty

3) Sour

4) Hot (Chilly)

5) Astringent

6) Bitter

It has been observed that we are avoiding more and more the last two types of taste with the result that it upsets the digestive system and balance in our blood, thereby leading to a number of diseases, including cancer. These tastes nullify the effect of sweets and purify the blood. These two tastes increase the digestive power – the fire- and are like a starter in a car and therefore should be included in our diet.

101 Fast And Natural Weight Loss Tips

We take great care about the quality and quantity of coal or wood we put in the cooking furnace or fireplace. We should also give it enough air to burn properly. This enables the fire to give maximum of heat and reduce smoke and ashes to a minimum.

We should not forget that there is a similar fireplace in our stomach. We must think of the after-effects of the food and drink we take. The difference in the proportion of three basic elements of water, fire and wood in our body depends upon the food we eat.

As laymen, we should see that the fire in the stomach is well maintained and should be knowledgeable on the type of food that does not agree with us. We should, therefore, avoid such unsuitable foods. We must know that a particular food which may be good for certain people may not be suitable to others eg, curd/yoghurt, buttermilk, suitable to people having more elements of fire, would not be suitable to people having more elements of water in them.

101 Fast And Natural Weight Loss Tips

Recent experiments by nutrition experts in the U.S.A. have confirmed the findings of the Indian philosophy, that eating late and taking heavy foods after sunset, tends to slow down digestion and produces more fat and problems of stomach.

In Ayurveda, the Indian medical system, a detailed description of the after-effects of the different types of cereals, vegetables, spices, fruits, milk, curd, buttermilk, herbs, minerals, etc. is given. This shows a deep study and research over hundreds of years. Ayurveda describes minutely what food to eat, how to eat and when to eat.

101 Fast And Natural Weight Loss Tips

To maintain a good digestive system we should see that:

1) The food is well-cooked and eaten warm/hot.
2) The use of whole wheat and rice is adequate.
3) Reduce or avoid use of fine flour and polished rice.
4) Use of fried things should be reduced.
5) Enough buttermilk and curd should be included in the diet.
6) Enough vegetables, raw and cooked and seasonal fruits should be taken.
7) The food should be properly chewed.
8) A time gap of 5 to 7 hours must be kept between two meals.
9) The habit of eating or drinking liquids except water or buttermilk between the meals should be stringently controlled.
10) The stomach is also a machine and so it should be given rest of at least one or two meals a week. At that time, only fruits or fruit juices or boiled water may be taken.

101 Fast And Natural Weight Loss Tips

To satisfy our palate is one of the greatest enjoyments of life. Eat anything you like once in a while, but respect nature's signal, which is given in the form of belching. That is nature's way of saying "I'm full."

You should stop eating further at that point. It is a yellow signal like the one at the traffic lights. If that cannot be done, you must stop at the second signal, which is like a red light. If you continue eating even after the second signal, please note that you are inviting trouble. Necessary changes in the food, diet, should be made according to the changes in seasons.

Please observe the motto that the fire in the stomach should be well preserved and should remain capable of digesting the food you eat.

A liberal use of ginger, pepper, eatables of bitter taste, Sunbath, regular exercise etc. helps this fire. While cold water, cold drinks, ice cream etc. reduce the fire and increase the burden on the digestive system. Please note that Heat is Life while Cold is Death. Eat or drink accordingly.

Sprouted Pulses: This may be taken by all people uncooked, but mixed with sesame, groundnut, raw, cabbage, dates, dried grapes or a little jaggery are also good for them. Sprouted pulses are also very good for reducing weight. In that case the use of dates, dried grapes or jaggery should be avoided as far as possible.

Test of proper digestive power and proper eating: After the meals, you should feel energetic, light in body and capable of work – even running if necessary. If you feel heavy, sleepy or dull, it indicates overeating or fast eating or a weakened digestive system.

Chapter 10

Working Out

You may not like what I am about to say, but dieting alone will not help you to lose weight. You have to give your body the exercise it needs. As I mentioned earlier, a couple of centuries ago, people were involved in a lot of manual labor.

This gave their bodies all the exercise that was needed. But due to the changed life styles, most of us do not have to engage in strenuous work. Most of us sit in front of computers all day long or engage in other sedentary works.

101 Fast And Natural Weight Loss Tips

It is because of this that exercise becomes crucial for weight loss. Generally people do not gain weight till their early twenties. But once they cross the 25 mark, then visible signs of weight gain can be seen everywhere and in the mid section in particular.

There is something very important that you have to understand if you are really considering the possibility of losing weight. You will have to consciously give your body the required exercise that it needs for the weight loss to be really effective.

Watching your diet alone is not going to yield results unless it is coupled with proper exercise. You have to make a conscious effort for this. And the solution for this is a work out routine. This is the first point under this section and I think I should say it clearly one more time.

Chapter 11

Working Out...It Is Good For You

When we think about the life in the country, there is always something rosy about it. What is it that the people in the country have that we do not? When you ponder about it you find that those lucky souls eat good food, they work really hard, by work I mean real physical work and they have good night's sleep. Of course they do not have all the amenities and facilities that the city life has to offer.

101 Fast And Natural Weight Loss Tips

But the city life comes with a lot of strings attached. People in the cities are generally less healthy than the people in the country. One of the reasons is pollution of course but the other reason is because people in the city do not get enough exercise.

Now, when I talk about healthy bodies please make no mistake about what I am referring to. I am not talking about the Mr. Universe kind of body, the bodies that we see on WWF.

I am talking about people who are fit. And fitness and exercise are just two sides of the same coin. They both go hand in hand.

In order to stay fit you need exercise and in order to exercise you need to be fit. But just because you are not fit now, it does not mean that you should not exercise.

And just like that, just because you do not have any visible excess fat on your body right now, it does not mean that you need no exercise. Exercise is the best way to keep obesity, cardio vascular disorders, hypertension and all those lifestyle-related disorders under control.

101 Fast And Natural Weight Loss Tips

First of all let us get one point straight, exercise does not necessarily mean pumping metal. If you do have the time to go to a gymnasium everyday, then that is well and good.

But I suppose most of us do not have the time for a regular work out in a gym. So the other alternative is to do it at home of course.

But whether it is at home or at a multi-gym, there is something that I want to tell you. Whatever you are doing, you must try and do it regularly.

Consistency is very important for an exercise routine to have the desired effect on our body. Getting started is the easy part, it is sticking to a regular exercise routine that is difficult and this is what makes most people give up in between.

Most people get on to a beautiful start. They buy track suits and gym-wear, running shoes and a whole lot of other gear. Their first day at the gym is almost a celebration.

Then as the days go on, they find it increasingly difficult to meet the domestic and professional demands and so their routine slows down and finally comes to a complete workout burn out. In other words, they stop working out completely

It is a universal fact that the most chosen time for work outs is the evenings. If you can stick to work out in the evenings then it is well and good. But most of us find ourselves exhausted in the evenings. We find ourselves physically and mentally drained. And at that time our bodies will be just too tired for a work out.

The result is that after the first few days of working out, the interest just dwindles away. The other reason is that in the evenings a thousand and one things may crop up and then there is hardly time for a warm up. So it is best to set aside some time for exercise in the morning itself.

There are two advantages of setting apart time in the morning. The first advantage is that in the morning our bodies are fresh and full of energy. Now over here I want to make one point clear.

There is a popular misconception that exercise depletes the body of energy but the case is just the opposite. Exercise pumps up more blood through the different parts of the

101 Fast And Natural Weight Loss Tips

body and warms up the body, so in fact, after exercise we feel more charged and ready to face the challenges of the day.

The second advantage is that in the morning we can plan for the whole day without letting the exercise routine affect the rest of our activities.

What about those of us who have never worked out before? In such cases you might need to start off under the personal supervision of an instructor and that may require that you go to a gym. But what I would suggest is that there are two simple things that any one can do for which you do not need the help of any instructor.

You know what these are? They are walking and swimming. Any body can walk and those of you who know how to swim can swim. For these two activities you do not need much gear and experts say that these two exercises have no side effects and are excellent stress busters.

So in the morning wake up just half an hour earlier, put on your walking shoes and hit the roads. Most roads will be less crowded at this hour and less polluted too. It is a wonderful way to start a day.